# EAR PAIN

MEDICALLY DEALING WITH EAR PAIN

## DR. J. SIMON

Contents

## INTRODUCTION

Ear pain, also known as otalgia, is a common symptom that can result from a variety of underlying illnesses that affect the tissues surrounding the ear or the ear itself. The pain can range from mild discomfort to severe, acute agony, and it can be either temporary or chronic. Ear pain can be associated with disorders of the middle, inner, or outer ears and affect people of all ages.

The complex ear organ is responsible for maintaining balance and hearing. It consists of three parts: the inner ear, which contains the vestibular system for balance and the cochlea for hearing, the middle ear, which contains the eardrum and three small bones called ossicles. The ear canal and the visible part of the ear, known as the pinna, make up the outer ear.

Ear discomfort can be caused by a variety of factors, including infections, trauma, altered air pressure from diving or flying, impacted earwax, abnormalities of the temporomandibular joint (TMJ), dental issues, or pain referred from nearby structures. Sometimes, a more serious systemic illness such as sinusitis or throat infections can be indicated by ear pain.

To effectively manage and treat ear discomfort, it is imperative to pinpoint its exact cause. A medical evaluation by a healthcare professional, such as an ENT specialist, is frequently necessary to identify the underlying issue and determine the best course of treatment.

Earache, discomfort, fullness or pressure in the ear, hearing loss, ringing in the ears (tinnitus), and in rare cases, fluid leakage are commonly experienced in conjunction with ear pain. The course of treatment may involve warm compresses, ear drops, medication, or, in severe cases, surgery, depending on the underlying cause.

Those with severe or persistent ear pain, especially if it is accompanied by other unsettling symptoms, should consult a doctor immediately in order to treat the underlying issue and relieve discomfort.

# CHAPTER ONE

## The Anatomy of the Ear

The intricate ear is responsible for both hearing and maintaining balance. Its three main divisions are the middle ear, inner ear, and outer ear.

**Outside Ear:**

The visible part of the ear, known as the outer ear, is made up of:

Sound waves are collected and directed into the ear canal by the external, cartilaginous structure called the pinna (auricle).

The external auditory canal, sometimes referred to as the ear canal, is a tube-like structure that extends from the pinna to the eardrum. It makes it easier for the middle ear to receive sound waves.

**Midline Ear:**

Behind the eardrum is the air-filled middle ear. It consists of:

The tympanic membrane, sometimes referred to as the eardrum, is a thin structure that vibrates in response to sound waves. It separates the outer ear from the middle ear.

Ossicles: The three small bones (malleus, incus, and stapes) in the eardrum magnify sound waves that are then transmitted to the inner ear.

The eustachian tube is a tiny tube that connects the back of the throat to the middle ear. It makes middle ear air pressure equalization and fluid drainage easier.

**Inner Ear:**

The complex architecture of the inner ear contributes to both hearing and balance. It includes:

The organ that converts sound waves into electrical signals that are sent to the brain for interpretation is the fluid-filled, spiral-shaped cochlea.

The vestibular system controls balance and spatial orientation. It is made up of semicircular canals and otolith organs.

Anatomical structures filled with fluid that detect head rotation are called semicircular canals.

Otolith Organs: The uterus and saccule sense head position and linear acceleration.

When combined, these components aid in the processes of hearing and balancing. Sound waves enter the ear through the outer ear and travel to the eardrum. The eardrum sends vibrations to the cochlea in the inner ear, which amplify and transfer the signals through the ossicles. The cochlea converts these vibrations into electrical signals, which are then sent to the brain for interpretation via the auditory nerve.

In addition to helping with hearing, the vestibular system in the inner ear also assists with maintaining balance by detecting changes in head position and movement. This knowledge is crucial for preserving equilibrium and coordinating bodily movements.

An understanding of ear anatomy is necessary for the diagnosis and treatment of conditions that may affect hearing or balance. Among other symptoms, otitis media, middle, or inner ear disorders can cause vertigo, ear pain, hearing loss, or balance issues. Medical professionals, like ENT specialists, can use this information to address ear-related problems and provide appropriate treatment.

### Common Causes of Ear Pain

Ear pain can be caused by a number of underlying conditions that affect the ear or nearby structures. Ascertaining the exact cause is necessary for efficient administration. Here are a few common causes of ear pain:

**Otitis media:**

inflammation or middle ear infection, often with fluid accumulation. Ear pain, hearing loss, and fever are possible side effects of this illness.

Otitis externa, also referred to as swimmer's ear

infection or inflammation of the ear canal, usually caused by the ear's retention of moisture. It may cause discharge, redness, swelling, and ear pain.

**The Eustachian Tube's Function:**

a compromised Eustachian tube, which could lead to an irregular middle ear pressure. This may cause ear pain and fullness in the ears.

**Earwax blockage:**

A buildup of earwax clogging the ear canal. Hearing loss, ear pain, and fullness in the ears could come from this.

**Inflammation of the sinus:**

The condition known as sinus inflammation impacts the sinuses near the ear. Sinusitis-related pain that is referred to the ears can cause ear pain.

**Temporomandibular Joint (TMJ) Disorders:**

jaw joint dysfunction, which may cause facial, ear, and jaw pain. TMJ problems can result from teeth grinding, jaw misalignment, and jaw clenching.



Referred pain to the ears may be the consequence of tooth infections or jaw-related dental problems.

**Strange Object in the Ear:**

The ear may become inflamed, painful, or even damaged when foreign objects are inserted into the ear canal.

**Changes in Air Pressure:**

Abrupt variations in air pressure, like those experienced while diving or flying in an aircraft, can cause ear pain. This is known as barotrauma.

## Trauma or Injury:

Physical trauma or direct blows to the ear can cause pain and possibly damage to the ear structures.

## Anomalous infections:

Ear infections in the middle, inner, or outer ears can cause pain. Either bacteria or viruses could be the source of these infections.

## Pain Assigned:

One could feel anxiety in the ear from nearby structures like the throat or jaw. For example, a throat infection or dental issue could be the cause of an earache.

**Nerve pain, or neuralgia:**

Conditions that affect the nerves surrounding the ear, such as trigeminal neuralgia, can cause sharp, shooting pain.

**TMJ-related migraines:**

One sign of migraines associated with TMJ dysfunction is ear pain.

**Extensions:**

Tumors in or near the ear, like acoustic neuromas, are rare causes of ear pain.

It is important to remember that severe or persistent ear pain needs to be assessed and diagnosed by a medical professional, especially if it coexists with other symptoms like fever, discharge, or hearing loss. The best course of action will depend on the underlying cause of the earache.



There are often several auxiliary symptoms that can be used in conjunction with otalgia, or ear pain, to identify the underlying cause. The specific features of ear pain may vary depending on the underlying causes.

**The following are typical signs and symptoms of ear pain:**

**A throbbing or numb pain**

People may experience a sharp, stabbing pain or a dull, persistent ear ache.

**Heart-stopping Emotion:**

Some people report having a throbbing or pulsating sensation in their ears.

**Radiation Anguish:**

There are several nearby areas where ear pain can radiate, including the jaw, throat, and side of the face.

**Increased Soreness When Moving the Jaw:**

Abnormalities of the temporomandibular joint (TMJ) may exacerbate ear pain during speaking or chewing.

# CHAPTER TWO

**Pain During Swallowing:**

Tonsillitis or throat infections can cause severe ear pain that gets worse when you swallow.

**Hearing Loss:**

Ear pain may be associated with permanent or temporary hearing loss.

**Tinnitus, or "ringing in the ears":**

Some people may report a ringing, buzzing, or humming sound in the affected ear.

**Fluid seepage or overflow:**

Otitis media or other disorders may cause pus, blood, or liquid to pour out of the ear canal.

**Redness or Swelling:**

Both inflammation and infection can result in ear swelling and redness.

**Itching Sensation:**

A sensation of tickling or itching in the ear is possible, particularly if you have otitis externa, often known as swimmer's ear.

**Ear Fullness or Pressure:**

People may feel as though their ears are full or compressed, especially if there is a buildup of fluid.

**An increase in temperature:**

There are situations when fever and ear infections are related.

**Issues with Stability:**

Diseases or infections of the inner ear can cause dizziness or problems with balance.

**Experiencing nausea or vomiting:**

Especially if it's linked to a condition like labyrinthitis, severe ear pain might induce nausea or vomiting.

**Pain Reacting to External Pressure:**

Applying external pressure, such as pushing on the earlobe, may exacerbate the pain in certain situations.

It's important to keep in mind that a variety of conditions, including dental disorders, trouble with the temporomandibular joint (TMJ), impacted earwax, sinus infections, ear infections (otitis media or externa), and even pain transmitted from surrounding tissues, can cause ear pain. When determining the cause of the ear pain, it can be helpful to consider the length of the discomfort, the presence of any associated risk factors, and the existence of any further symptoms.

If there are any indications of chronic or severe ear discomfort, it is best to get medical help for a thorough examination and diagnosis. An ENT specialist, for example, is a medical professional who may help identify the underlying cause and recommend the best course of action.

To determine the best course of action and identify the underlying cause of ear discomfort, a comprehensive examination is necessary for diagnosis and evaluation. Medical practitioners, which often include ENT specialists, employ a combination of physical examination, taking a patient's history, and ordering additional diagnostic tests as necessary. When diagnosing and treating ear pain, the following steps are essential:

**Background Information on Health:**

The medical practitioner will begin by taking a complete medical history, during which they will question about the onset and duration of the ear pain, any concomitant symptoms, recent illnesses, exposure to loud noises, recent travel, and any history of ear infections or injuries.

## An explanation for the discomfort in the ears

Patients will be asked to describe the nature of their pain, including if it is throbbing, dull, or sharp, whether it has migrated to other areas, and any potential causes or relief sources.

**Associated Symptoms:**

Concomitant symptoms, such as fever, vertigo, tinnitus (ear ringing), hearing loss, and ear discharge, will be the subject of data collection.

**Looking into the ears:**

An otoscope will be used to check the eardrum, external ear canal, and other structures during a thorough examination of the ear. Redness, swelling, discharge, or anomalies in the ears can all provide important diagnostic indications.

## Assessment of Auditory Processing

Tests of hearing can be performed to evaluate any abnormalities in auditory function. This can entail tympanometry, audiometry, or tuning fork testing.

## Using a Nasopharyngeal Exam

The healthcare professional may examine the nasopharynx and throat to assess for symptoms of infections or other diseases that may be contributing to ear pain.

**Imaging Studies:**

In some circumstances, imaging examinations may be recommended to see the interior components of the ear or discover any underlying abnormalities. This can include:

Computed Tomography (CT) Scan: Provides comprehensive images of the ear structures and adjacent areas.

Magnetic Resonance Imaging (MRI): Useful for examining soft tissues and structures in and around the ear.

**Specialized Testing:**

Based on the suspected reason of ear pain, specialist testing may be ordered. As an illustration:

Tympanocentesis: A method to collect fluid from the middle ear for laboratory investigation.

Allergy Testing: To discover probable allergens leading to ear pain.

**Tinnitus Assessment:**

If tinnitus is present, additional examinations may be undertaken to examine the nature and impact of the ringing or buzzing noises.

**Consultations:**

Referral to other experts, such as a dentist or neurologist, may be considered if the reason of ear pain extends beyond ENT-related disorders.

**Observation and Succession:**

Continuous monitoring of symptoms and follow-up sessions are crucial to track the course of treatment and make modifications as needed.

The diagnosis technique is personalized depending on the patient's specific symptoms, medical history, and examination findings. Prompt and correct diagnosis is critical for defining the best effective treatment plan and addressing any underlying issues contributing to ear pain. If ear discomfort is severe, chronic, or combined with worrying symptoms, persons should seek quick medical assistance for a comprehensive evaluation.



The therapy of ear discomfort relies on the underlying reason. It's crucial to precisely assess the specific condition leading to the ear ache before executing a targeted treatment plan. Here are common therapeutic approaches for different causes of ear pain:

**Ear Infections (Otitis Media or Otitis Externa):**

Bacterial Infections: Antibiotic medicines are recommended to treat bacterial ear infections.

Viral Infections: Viral infections are normally handled with supportive treatment, including pain medications and rest.

Pain Management: Over-the-counter pain medications such as acetaminophen or ibuprofen can help decrease discomfort.

**The Eustachian Tube's Function:**

Nasal Decongestants: Decongestant medicines can help relieve congestion and enhance Eustachian tube function.

Nasal Steroids: In some circumstances, nasal steroid sprays may be prescribed to relieve inflammation.

**Impacted Earwax:**

Ear Drops: Earwax softening drops may be used to help soften and simplify the evacuation of impacted earwax.

Irrigation: Ear irrigation, performed by a healthcare expert, may be necessary to eliminate obstinate earwax.

## Temporomandibular Joint (TMJ) Disorders:

Pain Medications: Over-the-counter pain medicines may be given to alleviate discomfort.

Jaw Exercises: Physical therapy exercises to improve jaw function and lessen pain.

## Sinus Infections or Allergies:

Antibiotics: If a bacterial infection is present, antibiotics may be recommended.

Decongestants: Medications that relieve sinus congestion.

Antihistamines: If allergies are leading to ear pain.

**Tinnitus:**

Management of Underlying Cause: Addressing the underlying cause of tinnitus, such as hearing loss or exposure to loud noises.

Counseling and Support: Counseling or support groups for persons having bothersome tinnitus.

**Strange Object in the Ear:**

Removal: Safe removal of the foreign object by a healthcare expert.

**Migraines or Headaches:**

Migraine Medications: Medications prescribed to manage migraines and accompanying symptoms.

**Barotrauma (Pressure Changes):**

Pressure Equalization Techniques: Equalizing pressure during changes in altitude or scuba diving.

Decongestants: Medications to relieve nasal congestion and aid in pressure equalization.

**Labyrinthitis or Vestibular Disorders:**

Vestibular Rehabilitation: Exercises to enhance balance and minimize symptoms.

drugs: Antiemetic or antivertigo drugs to alleviate dizziness.

**TMJ-related migraines:**

TMJ Treatment: Addressing underlying TMJ disorders with dental procedures, physical therapy, or splints.

It's crucial to remember that self-diagnosis and self-treatment may not be suitable, especially if the cause of ear pain is unknown. Seeking quick medical attention is advisable for a comprehensive evaluation and proper management. Individuals should follow the suggestions of healthcare professionals and finish prescribed therapies for the greatest outcomes.

## DIY Solutions & Self-Treatment

While it's vital to check with a healthcare expert for a proper diagnosis and treatment of ear discomfort, there are certain home remedies and self-care practices that may provide relief for minor cases or while waiting for medical assistance.



**Warm Compress:**

Applying a warm compress to the afflicted ear might help ease pain and reduce inflammation. Ensure the compress is not too hot to avoid burning.

**Over-the-Counter Pain Relievers:**

Non-prescription pain medications, such as acetaminophen or ibuprofen, can help alleviate discomfort and reduce inflammation. Follow the indicated dosage.



## Consuming lots of water

Staying well-hydrated can boost overall health and may help ease symptoms linked with certain causes of ear pain.

**Ear Drops:**

Over-the-counter ear drops, meant to soften earwax, may be used to help manage impacted earwax. Follow the instructions on the product.

**Avoid Inserting Objects:**

Avoid placing cotton swabs or any other things into the ear canal, since this might push earwax farther down or cause harm.

**Rest:**

Getting appropriate rest and avoiding activities that may increase symptoms, such as loud noises or excessive jaw movement, might be beneficial.

**Steam Inhalation:**

Inhaling steam from a bowl of hot water may help relieve congestion and lessen symptoms linked with sinus infections or nasal congestion.

**Elevate Head During Sleep:**

Elevating the head with an extra cushion during sleep may help decrease pressure in the ears.

**Chewing Gum:**

Chewing gum can help equalize pressure in the ears, particularly during changes in altitude.

**Avoid Smoking and Secondhand Smoke:**

Smoke can irritate the ears, so avoiding smoking and exposure to secondhand smoke is recommended.

**Hydrogen Peroxide Solution:**

For impacted earwax, a few drops of a mixture of equal parts hydrogen peroxide and water may be used to soften earwax. Consult with a healthcare expert before attempting this.

**Maintain a Nutritious Diet:**

A well-balanced diet helps support general health, including the health of the ears.

It's crucial to note that these home remedies are not a substitute for professional medical advice, diagnosis, or treatment. If ear discomfort persists, intensifies, or is accompanied by other troubling symptoms, finding early medical assistance is vital. Home remedies are generally appropriate for addressing mild symptoms, but the underlying cause should be addressed by a healthcare professional for successful and safe therapy.

## Coping Strategies and Lifestyle Modifications

Coping with ear discomfort needs a combination of lifestyle modifications and tactics to reduce symptoms and manage the underlying reasons. Here are some coping tactics and lifestyle adaptations for ear pain:

**Follow Medical Advice:**

Adhere to the recommendations and treatment regimens provided by healthcare specialists. If prescribed drugs, take them as advised.

**Practice Good Ear Hygiene:**

Avoid introducing items, such as cotton swabs, into the ear canal. Clean the outer ear carefully with a washcloth. If earwax is an issue, visit a healthcare expert for safe removal.

**Protect Your Ears:**

Use ear protection, such as earplugs or earmuffs, in noisy locations or during activities with high noise levels to prevent further damage.

**Avoid Smoke Exposure:**

Minimize exposure to cigarette smoke and other environmental toxins, as they might irritate the ears.

**Manage Your Tension:**

Practice stress-reduction practices, such as deep breathing, meditation, or yoga, as stress can add to tension and increase symptoms.

**Maintain a Nutritious Diet:**

Consume a well-balanced diet rich in vitamins and minerals to promote general health, including ear health.

**Retain Hydration:**

Drink a proper amount of water to maintain hydration, which can contribute to general well-being.

**Modify Sleeping Positions:**

Elevate the head with an extra cushion during sleep to decrease pressure in the ears, especially if having congestion.

**Use Humidifiers:**

Humidifiers can add moisture to the air, which may be beneficial for persons with dry or sensitive ears.

**Limit Exposure to Allergens:**

Minimize exposure to irritants that may lead to ear pain, such as pollen, dust, or pet dander.

**Practice Jaw Exercises:**

If ear pain is connected with temporomandibular joint (TMJ) disorders, do gentle jaw exercises advised by a healthcare expert.

**Avoid Loud Noises:**

Limit exposure to loud noises or use ear protection in instances where loud sounds are unavoidable.

**Monitor and Manage Tinnitus:**

If having tinnitus, implement techniques to manage and cope with the sounds. This may involve using white noise devices or engaging in activities that distract from the noise.

# CHAPTER THREE

**Remain Up to Date:**

Educate yourself on the underlying cause of ear discomfort and work cooperatively with healthcare providers to manage and address symptoms.

**Seek Emotional Support:**

Share your experience with friends, family, or support groups to obtain emotional support and understanding.

It's crucial to personalize coping tactics to the precise source of ear pain and individual circumstances. Consultation with healthcare professionals, particularly ear, nose, and throat

(ENT) specialists, can guide suitable lifestyle modifications and coping methods for effective symptom management. If ear discomfort persists or worsens, seeking urgent medical assistance is necessary for further examination and intervention.

## Warning Signs and When to Get Help from a Doctor

While many cases of ear pain can be treated with home remedies or over-the-counter drugs, certain "red flags" suggest a need for quick medical intervention. If you have any of the following signs or symptoms combined with ear pain, seek medical assistance promptly:

**Extreme Pain:**

Intense or severe ear discomfort that is not alleviated by over-the-counter pain drugs.

**An increase in temperature:**

The appearance of a fever, especially if accompanied by additional symptoms like chills or sweating, may suggest an illness that requires medical treatment.

**Drainage or Discharge:**

Discharge of pus, blood, or clear fluid from the ear is a worrying indication and may suggest an infection or injury.

**Hearing Loss:**

Sudden or substantial hearing loss accompanied with ear pain demands quick medical intervention.

**Dizziness or Vertigo:**

Persistent dizziness or vertigo (a spinning sensation) may be indicative of inner ear disorders, such as labyrinthitis.

**Facial Weakness or Paralysis:**

If ear pain is accompanied by facial weakness or paralysis, it may be a sign of a more serious ailment, such as Bell's palsy.

Swelling around the ear or on the face may signal an underlying condition that needs investigation.

**Neck Stiffness or Rigidity:**

Stiffness or rigidity in the neck, especially if it is difficult to touch the chin to the chest, may be an indication of meningitis.

**Persistent or Recurrent Symptoms:**

If ear pain persists for more than a few days or recurs regularly, it's necessary to seek medical assessment to discover and address the underlying cause.

**Recent Injury or Trauma:**

If ear pain is the consequence of recent trauma or injury to the head or ear, get medical assistance to examine for possible damage.

**Persistent Tinnitus:**

Continuous or worsening tinnitus (ringing in the ears) should be checked by a healthcare expert.

**Recent Surgery:**

If you've recently undergone ear surgery and are experiencing new or increasing pain, contact your surgeon for help.

**Difficulty Swallowing:**

Difficulty swallowing or expanding the mouth wide may be indicative of a more serious issue and requires medical intervention.

**Pain Radiating to Jaw or Neck:**

If ear discomfort travels to the jaw or neck, it may be a sign of referred pain from other structures that need investigation.

**Development of Rash:**

If a rash develops around the ear or on the face, it may be associated to an infectious disease requiring medical attention.

If you experience any of these red signs or if you are confused about the severity of your symptoms, it's vital to seek medical assistance soon. Delaying care may lead to complications or impair the prompt therapy of underlying diseases. An evaluation by a healthcare professional, such as an ear, nose, and throat

(ENT) specialist, can assist diagnose the origin of ear pain and lead proper treatment.

## Ear Pain in Special Populations

Ear discomfort can afflict individuals across many age groups and populations, and particular groups may be more sensitive to specific causes of ear pain. Here are concerns for ear pain in particular populations:

**Infants and Young Children:**

Common Causes: Ear infections, teething, or foreign objects in the ear.

Symptoms: Irritability, pulling or straining at the ear, crying, fever, and difficulties sleeping.

Note: Infants and young children may not be able to explain their symptoms orally, making it vital for parents to notice behavioral changes.

**Children and Adolescents:**

Common Causes: Ear infections, swimmer's ear, foreign objects, or trauma.

Symptoms: Ear pain, hearing loss, ear discharge, and changes in behavior.

Note: Frequent exposure to water, such as during swimming, can raise the risk of swimmer's ear.

**Pregnant Women:**

Common Causes: Changes in hormone levels, increased blood flow, and possible infections.

Symptoms: Ear pain, alterations in hearing, or greater susceptibility to infections.

Note: Pregnancy-related hormonal changes can increase the susceptibility to ear infections.

**Older Adults:**

Common Causes: Hearing loss, age-related changes in the ear, and increased risk of earwax impaction.

Symptoms: Gradual hearing loss, tinnitus, and balance difficulties.

Note: Presbycusis, age-related hearing loss, is a common problem among older persons.

**People who have diabetes:**

Common Causes: Increased risk of ear infections, poor wound healing, and neuropathy.

Symptoms: Chronic ear infections, sluggish healing of ear injuries, and probable hearing loss.

Note: Diabetes can damage the immune system and the body's ability to fight infections.

**Individuals with Allergies:**

Common Causes: Allergic rhinitis, sinus congestion, and eustachian tube dysfunction.

Symptoms: Ear pressure, pain, and alterations in hearing during allergy seasons.

Note: Allergies can contribute to congestion and inflammation in the ear and nasal passages.

**Individuals with Immunocompromised Conditions:**

Common Causes: Increased susceptibility to infections, including ear infections.

Symptoms: Persistent or recurrent ear infections, poor recovery from ear-related disorders.

Note: Weakened immune systems can render patients more prone to numerous illnesses.

**Individuals with Neurological Disorders:**

Common Causes: Increased risk of vestibular diseases, which may contribute to dizziness or imbalance.

Symptoms: Vertigo, unbalance, and coordination problems.

Note: Neurological problems may impair the functioning of the inner ear.

It's vital to note that persons in specific demographics may encounter distinct issues and considerations linked to ear pain. Any persistent or severe ear discomfort, especially in these special populations, should be checked by a healthcare professional for a complete diagnosis and proper management.

## CONCLUSION

Ear discomfort can be a painful symptom that develops from several underlying reasons. From basic ailments like ear infections to more difficult conditions such as neurological abnormalities, recognizing the particular cause is vital for effective care. Seeking immediate medical assistance is vital, especially when red flags such as significant discomfort, fever, or drainage are present.

In many circumstances, ear pain can be controlled with appropriate medical measures, including drugs, ear drops, or, in some cases, surgical operations. Lifestyle adjustments and self-care practices, such as keeping excellent ear cleanliness and protecting the ears from loud noises, can also contribute to overall ear health.

It's crucial to remember that ear discomfort is not a one-size-fits-all illness, and the approach to diagnosis and treatment should be personalized to the individual's specific symptoms, medical history, and any underlying health concerns.

Regular check-ups with healthcare professionals, particularly ear, nose, and throat specialists, can contribute to the early detection and management of ear-related disorders.

If you or someone you know feels persistent or severe ear discomfort, especially when accompanied by red flags or troubling symptoms, don't hesitate to seek medical treatment. A healthcare practitioner can do a comprehensive assessment, arrange diagnostic tests if necessary, and prescribe an appropriate treatment plan to address the underlying cause and alleviate symptoms.

Remember, the material presented here is for general informational purposes and is not a substitute for professional medical advice.

Always consult with a trained healthcare provider for specialized guidance and care. Take care of your ears, and prioritize your ear health to guarantee optimal well-being.

**THE END**